PLANTS, PERFORMANCE
AND THE ENDOCANNABINOID SYSTEM

21ST CENTURY SPORTS MEDICINE

DON MCLAUGHLIN
& DOUG BROWN

Contents

Acknowledgments		5
Introduction		7
1	A Ski Pro's Story	11
2	Hemp as Uber Adaptogen	15
3	What is the Endocannabinoid System?	19
4	CBD Isolate vs. Full-Spectrum Hemp Oil	25
5	Phytocannabinoids For Potent Energy and Endurance	29
6	CBD for Stress-Busting and Anxiety Reduction	35
7	CBD For Deep Sleep	41
8	CBD For Beating Inflammation	45
9	The CBD Advantage for Athletes	51
10	Beyond CBD	55
Plant Power Case Studies		57
Conclusion		61
Learn About the Authors		63
Notes		65

Copyright © 2019 by Don McLaughlin

All rights reserved. No part of this book may be used or reproduced in any manner whatsoever without written permission from the publisher and copyright holder, except in the case of brief quotations embodied in critical reviews and certain other noncommercial uses permitted by copyright law.

ISBN 978-1-72949-552-0

Statements made herein have not been evaluated by the Food and Drug Administration (FDA). The efficacy of the materials and/or products discussed in this publication have not been confirmed by FDA-approved research. The information provided herein, along with any of the products or ingredients mentioned, are not intended to diagnose, treat, cure or prevent any disease. All information presented here is not meant as a substitute for or alternative to information from health care practitioners. Please consult your healthcare professional about potential interactions or other possible complications before using any product. The Federal Food and Cosmetic Act requires this notice.

Acknowledgments

FIRST, I want to thank my co-author, Doug Brown, without whom this book would not exist. Doug worked tirelessly to shape the contents of this book into a compelling narrative about the positive impact of these powerful plants. Thank you, Doug, for your persistence, dogged research, and deft writing throughout. I also want to thank certain contributors to this book, including Eric Henderson, Jim McAlpine, Kyle Turley, and Avery Collins. Thank you for making the time to share your individual journeys, and in so doing raise more and more awareness about the miraculous power of a very special plant. Finally, I want to thank my cousin, Sean McCabe, whose own use of hemp and other plant extracts during his recovery from a near-fatal head injury continually inspired us as we wrote this book.

Introduction

THE STORY behind this book begins in 2012, after I hit my lowest point in life. I was a forty-three-year-old burned-out CEO, struggling to turn things around in a multi-million-dollar tech consulting and services firm I had cofounded several years earlier. The business served legal departments in the Fortune 500, and I worked constantly, suffering prolonged anxiety, severe bouts of depression, and sleepless nights while working on complex, high-profile legal matters that often hit the front pages of the national newspapers.

The pressure was intense, and at times the stress was nearly unbearable. During particularly bad episodes, it felt as if I were trapped in a long, dark hallway from which I could not escape. Prescription anti-depressants helped, but I was constantly exhausted, living on a roller-coaster of caffeine to speed me up and alcohol to slow me down.

I finally hit bottom in late 2012, and after what I can only describe as a spiritual awakening, I reemerged with more passion and commitment than ever before. I overhauled my diet and began regular high-intensity exercise. The business began to flourish.

Around this time, I became a high-altitude, ultra-endurance trail runner, running fifty and then a hundred miles. And all of this happened in my mid-forties, with zero long-distance running experience. What could explain this transformation? I had no running pedigree, no coach, and in the past, I'd hated running. In fact, I was kicked off my high school cross-country team for being a poor, disinterested runner. But for some reason, running—particularly high-altitude mountain trail running—became a lifeline to me in my mid-forties.

Along the way, I investigated anything I thought might support my recovery and sustain this newfound energy. I explored and experimented with everything from ancient, natural healing methods to the latest, most advanced bio-hacking techniques. As a Colorado resident, I began to read articles in the Denver Post about the emerging legalization of cannabis, and about its medicinal or therapeutic uses. This surprised me—as a former assistant district attorney, I had only witnessed the negative aspects of cannabis.

But as I researched more and more, I discovered that some athletes and other high performers were starting to use an extract of the non-psychoactive form of cannabis (hemp) to deal with stress, and promote energy and recovery. I learned quickly that while hemp and marijuana come from the same plant, oil extracted from hemp delivers a huge range of health benefits without the "high" of marijuana.

So, for the same reasons as those athletes, I started using it. I found that I was sleeping better. I discovered a new sense of calm, and was able to manage stress far more effectively than before. I began looking after my health in a variety of ways: I overhauled my diet, weaned myself off the meds, and started a consistent meditation practice. I also began experimenting with other plant extracts that I learned might work more effectively in combination with hemp. My mental outlook, overall energy, and endurance soared. It felt like I had found the fountain of youth. I started running long distances, largely injury-free, and I haven't stopped since.

It was high above Aspen, Colorado—during the Audi Power of Four race, one of my mountain ultra-trail running events—that I was inspired to write this book. I was heading into the ninth hour of that race, having climbed and descended over 12,000 feet on miles of muddy trail, through rain and hail, when something powerful came over me. It prodded me both to share my journey (as I've done briefly here), and to raise awareness, shining a spotlight on the hemp plant, which helped turn things around so dramatically for me, and other plants that have helped me. I hope this book opens your eyes to the benefits of the hemp plant and provides you with some inspiration to attempt greater and greater challenges—challenges that will take you to the next level in life.

1 A SKI PRO'S STORY

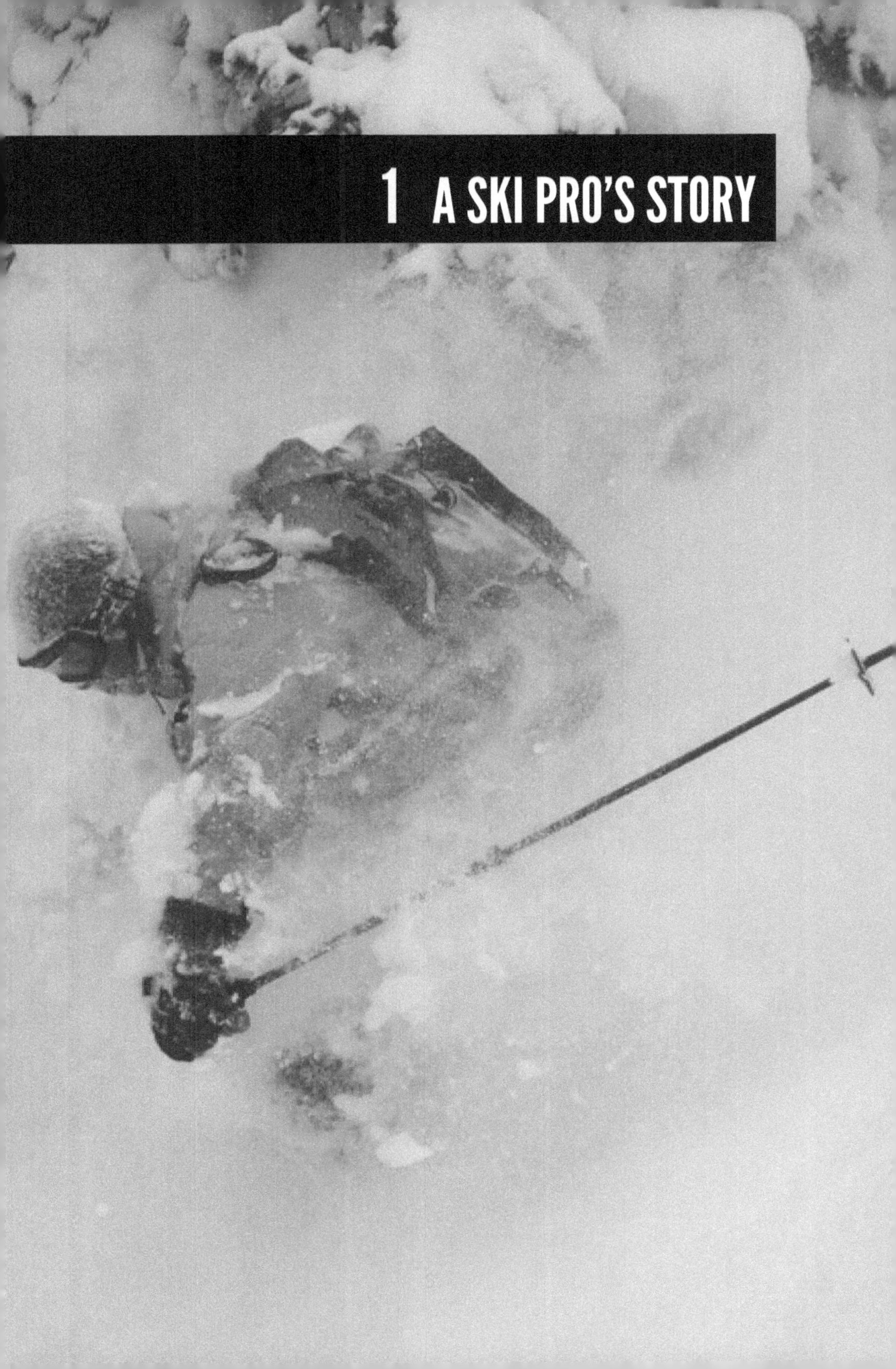

A Ski Pro's Story

THE SLOPE on the Alaskan glacier was steep, the line tight, when former ski pro and snowsports legend Eric Henderson[1] fell, tumbling down the mountain head over heels and breaking his neck. That dive ended his professional ski career, but Henderson, known as "Hende," recovered and is back on his boards again; he even tackled the same line on that glacier five years later. Filmmakers shot the adventure and turned it into a movie.[2]

He credits rehabilitation work, lots of exercise, a healthy diet, and a positive outlook for his recovery—and his secret weapon for recovery, CBD.

"Skiing was my life for decades, and as soon as I understood that I could recover, I began researching all of the strategies for nursing myself back to health," said Hende, who now lives in Boulder and runs Meteorite, a mountain sports PR agency. "At the time, CBD[3] wasn't widely known, but some of my mountain jock pals swore by it. I started taking CBD supplements, and I felt my aches and pains soften. My sleep deepened. My anxiety dropped. It wasn't some sort of magic pill, but I think it was an important part of my recovery. And now, I use CBD to help improve my skiing, trail running and training."

Hende is not alone. As CBD is embraced by the mainstream, athletes in particular are turning to natural compounds to help manage inflammation and pain, to boost energy, and to help them fully embrace downtime—they ratchet down stress and anxiety, sinking into the deep, satisfying sleep that is key for athletic recovery.

"Athletes of all stripes are turning to CBD, in larger and larger numbers every month," said Jim McAlpine,[4] the founder of the 420 Games[5] and the most prominent advocate for CBD and athletics in the nation. Jim is also active with Athletes For Care,[6] a cannabis-championing nonprofit representing a wide range of professional athletes, including former NFL stars Jim McMahon and Jake Plummer. "With cannabis, recovery from training and competition is key for many athletes, but athletes now are also using it to improve overall performance. Lately, more and more athletes in hard-hitting sports like football are also using CBD prophylactically, as a neuro-protector. They believe it helps them deal better with hits to the brain. We are all thankful for the social and scientific progress that is being made with cannabis in the world. For athletes, it is a treasure."

The turn to plant power is not limited to CBD or to athletes: research into interactions between plant properties and the human body is leading to a wide range of powerful insights. Botanicals, adaptogens, and the natural compounds found in ashwagandha, turmeric, boswellia, magnesium, milk thistle, and Vitamin D are being tapped by athletes and others wrestling with stress and fatigue to persevere through their struggles and triumph as never before. But first, let's turn our attention to the master of all adaptogens, hemp.

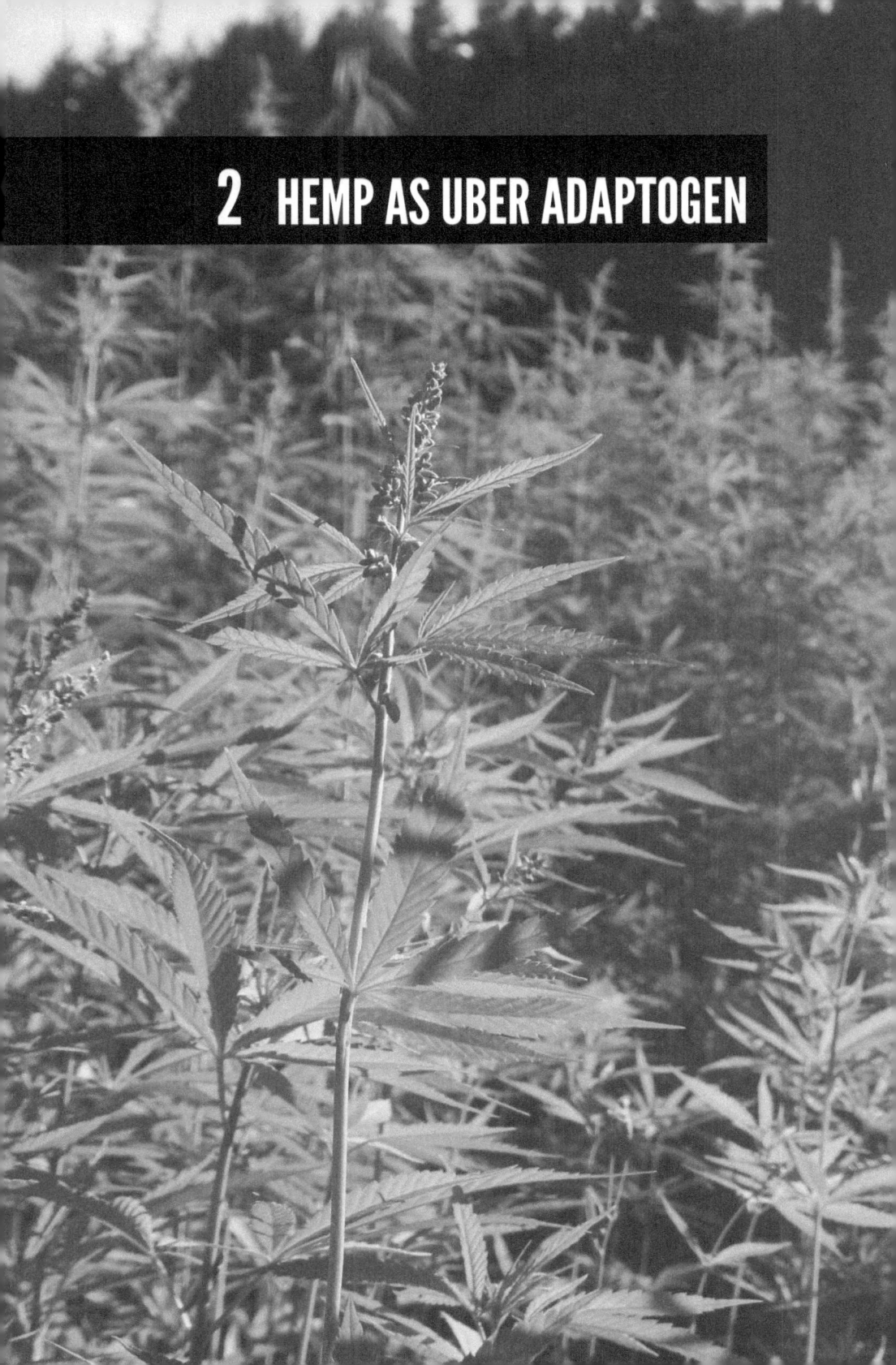

2 HEMP AS UBER ADAPTOGEN

Hemp as Uber Adaptogen

What Is Hemp-Derived CBD and How Does It Work?

RESEARCH into the *cannabis sativa* plant led scientists to one of the more interesting health-related discoveries in recent decades: the endocannabinoid system, which scientists first encountered in 1992. This fascinating system serves the body in different ways, but one common thread is its role in helping to achieve homeostasis[7] —the system acts like a team of mechanics to the body's machinery, spending every moment toiling to make sure that all the parts are properly oiled, that timing belts are spinning smoothly, pistons are firing with precision, and fuel is efficiently distributed. The endocannabinoid system is part of what makes the inner workings of a human body "hum," and phytocannabinoids play an important role in helping the endocannabinoid system achieve that wonderful hum.

What Is Non-Psychoactive Hemp Oil (and its biggest constituent part - CBD)?

Not so long ago, no one understood phytocannabinoids, not even the best-known, CBD (cannabidiol). CBD is one of many natural compounds found in the cannabis plant and the one most widely recognized and celebrated for its benefits. Importantly, the cannabis plant has two varieties, marijuana and hemp. While marijuana and hemp come from the same *cannabis sativa* plant, marijuana includes high amounts of psychoactive compounds, including THC, while hemp plants do not. The key difference? CBD derived from hemp oil extract doesn't get you "high" like marijuana. For the purposes of this discussion, we'll be talking about CBD and other cannabinoids derived from non-psychoactive hemp oil.

What Are Phytocannabinoids?

More than a hundred natural cannabinoids have been identified in the hemp plant, many with significant therapeutic and performance benefits for a wide range of health conditions. Cannabinoids contained within plants are called phytocannabinoids. Some of the most recognized phytocannabinoids are cannabidiol (CBD), cannabichromene (CBC), cannabigerol (CBG), and cannabinol (CBN). These phytocannabinoids influence the body's endocannabinoid system.

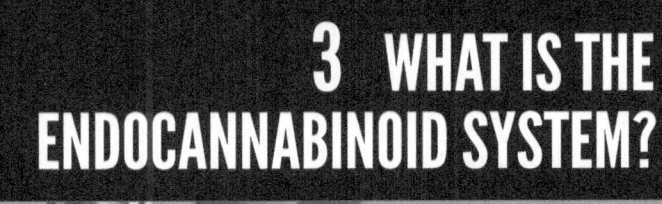

3 WHAT IS THE ENDOCANNABINOID SYSTEM?

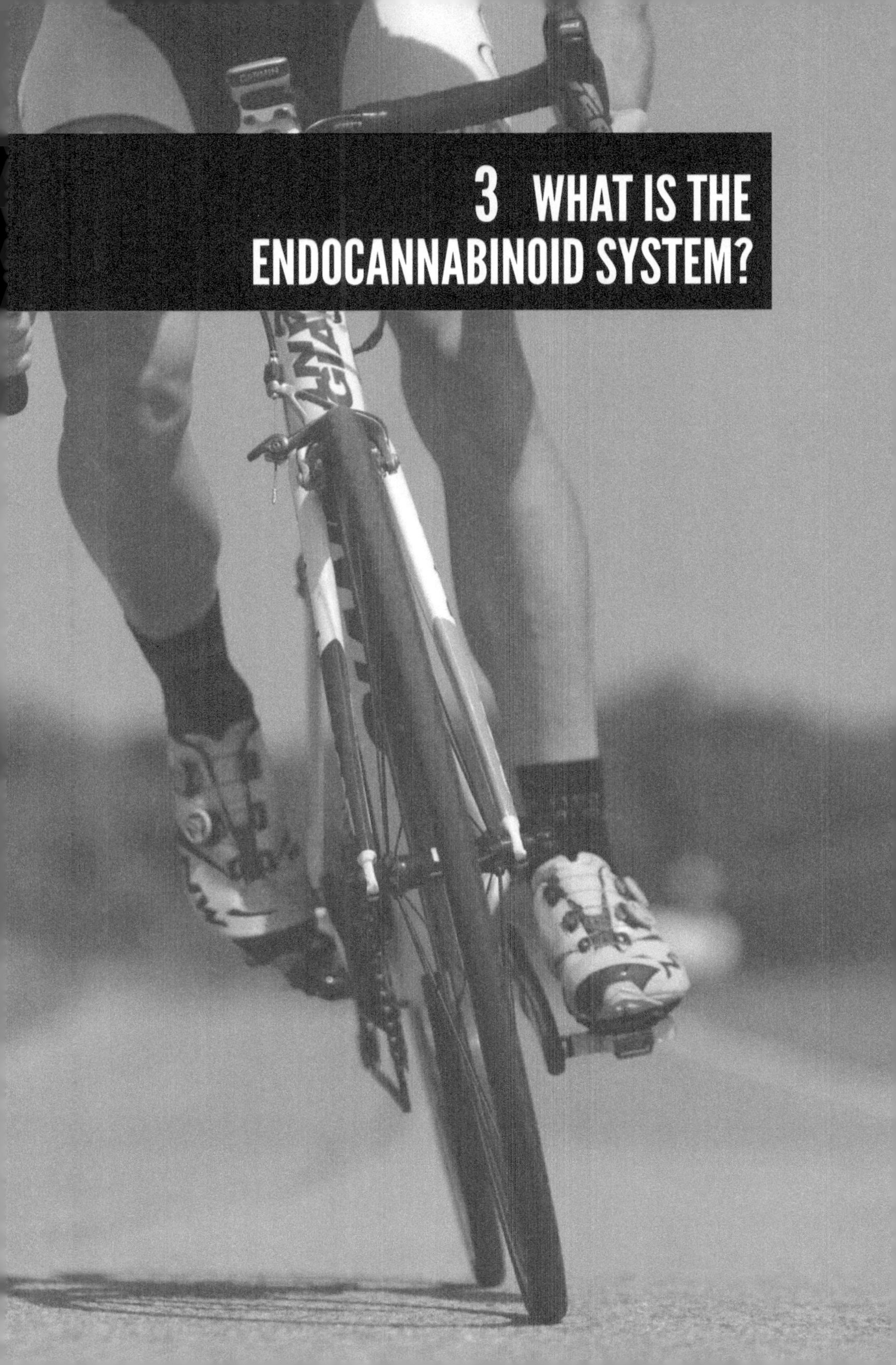

What Is the Endocannabinoid System?

SCIENTISTS discovered the endocannabinoid system (ECS)[8] in the early 1990s while studying the health impacts of cannabis. These studies showed that the ECS has key regulatory functions that help keep all physiological systems in balance. It was an extraordinary medical breakthrough, and the ECS is now considered one of the primary physiological systems in the human body.

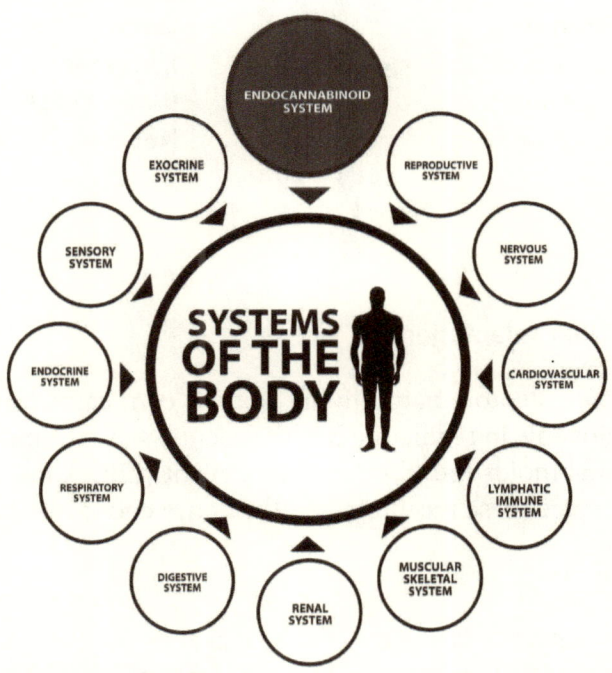

In short, the ECS is a system of neurotransmitters and receptors found within cells throughout the brain and body. Like all cellular receptors, these receptors accept certain "keys" found on various substances that allow those substances to enter the cell. Certain cell receptors that make up the ECS (CB1 and CB2 receptors) are highly concentrated in cells in specific regions such as the brain, the central nervous system, and the immune system. Scientists discovered that these receptors are capable of influencing all other physiological systems, and that the ECS is a primary mechanism for maintaining health and well-being—what's commonly referred to as "homeostasis."

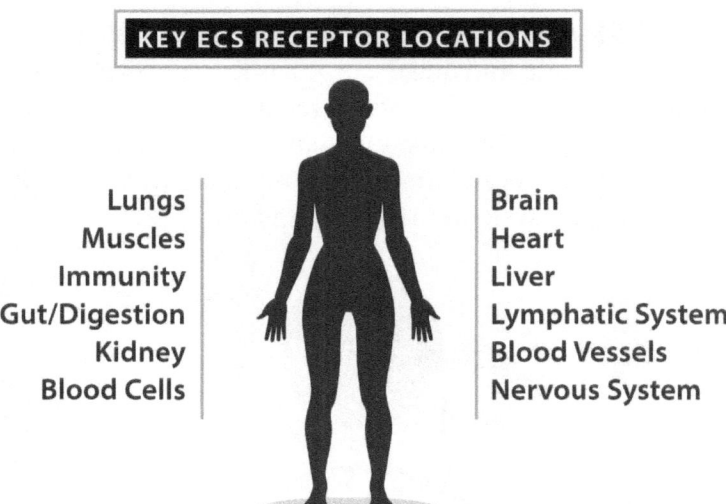

Hemp as Uber Adaptogen

While these receptors naturally make their own cannabinoids and play a major role in regulating health, scientists also discovered that phytocannabinoids found in the hemp plant (CBD, CBN, CBC and CBG) influence these receptors and the entire endocannabinoid system.

> *[W]ith its complex actions in our immune system, nervous system, and virtually all of the body's organs, the endocannabinoids are literally a bridge between body and mind. By understanding this system, we begin to see a mechanism that could connect brain activity and states of physical health and disease.*
>
> **University of Maryland medical researcher Dr. Bradley Alger**

The system's three key components are

> Cannabinoid receptors,[9] which behave like scouts for cells—they remain fixed on the surface of cells, monitoring what is going on around the cell. The receptors then relay their findings back to the inside of the cell. CBD, which is one of about 113 cannabinoids found in the hemp plant, interacts directly with these receptors; the communication between CBD and receptors is one of the foundations of CBD's effectiveness.

> Endocannabinoids,[10] the body's own homemade cannabinoids, which are essential for activating the receptors; without endocannabinoids, those lookouts—the receptors—would lose their effectiveness.

> Metabolic enzymes,[11] which help optimize the system by eliminating the endocannabinoids after they have performed their duties.

As University of Maryland medical researcher Dr. Bradley Alger writes in a 2013 scientific paper,[12] "With its complex actions in our immune system, nervous system, and virtually all of the body's organs, the endocannabinoids are literally a bridge between body and mind. By understanding this system, we begin to see a mechanism that could connect brain activity and states of physical health and disease."

How Does CBD Help Athletes?

For centuries, athletes have leveraged natural substances—everything from hunks of carbohydrate-dense bread to gulps of caffeine-abundant coffee to willow tree bark (a natural painkiller)—to enhance athletic performance.

The list of competition-approved athletic aids is long, but the most promising of all in the modern era are phytocannabinoids, newly discovered plant compounds that optimize performance through different, and novel, channels compared to substances like stimulants and painkillers. Phytocannabinoids, including CBD, augment the brain's ability to improve athletic performance while also delivering powerful benefits to the hard-charging body. And they achieve this kaleidoscopic range of tasks in both the body and the brain without the anxiety, jitters, and heart palpitations that stimulants produce or the long-term health risks and negative side effects of many analgesics. Ibuprofen, for example (used so frequently by athletes that it's been dubbed "vitamin I"), is known to cause liver damage, and has recently been tied to infertility in men).

And instead of producing a one-time effect—a quick jolt of energy or a bit of post-workout pain reduction— phytocannabinoids from hemp work synergistically within the body to produce long-lasting and sustainable health benefits in different key areas, many of which are of broad help to athletes engaged in rigorous training regimes and facing tough competition.

CBD's success among athletes also has major implications for anyone managing a stressful life—in other words, most human beings. Athletes face the same day-to-day life struggles as the rest of us, but they also confront the added challenges of extreme physical stress, which often leads to total breakdowns: physical, mental, and emotional. Athletes' increasing reliance on phytocannabinoids like CBD for overall support has echoes beyond the world of training and competition. If it's working for them, CBD offers potent benefits for just about everybody else.

The body-brain connection is central to CBD's positive impact on health. It has many advantages for athletes, according to recent research: CBD activates serotonin receptors,[13] diminishing anxiety and improving sleep; it influences a family of receptors called TRPV that regulate pain and inflammation[14] (helpful not just for recovery, but for handling pain while competing and training); it boosts the levels of something called adenosine in the brain, which is important for cardiovascular function, coronary blood flow, oxygen consumption, and inflammation. In addition, research shows that phytocannabinoids help optimize the body's consumption and distribution of fuel—in other words, they enhance energy. This is why hemp-derived CBD promises to be the next big game changer in the world of natural health supplements. But the question arises: is all hemp-derived CBD created equal? The answer: a resounding no.

4 CBD ISOLATE VS. FULL-SPECTRUM HEMP OIL

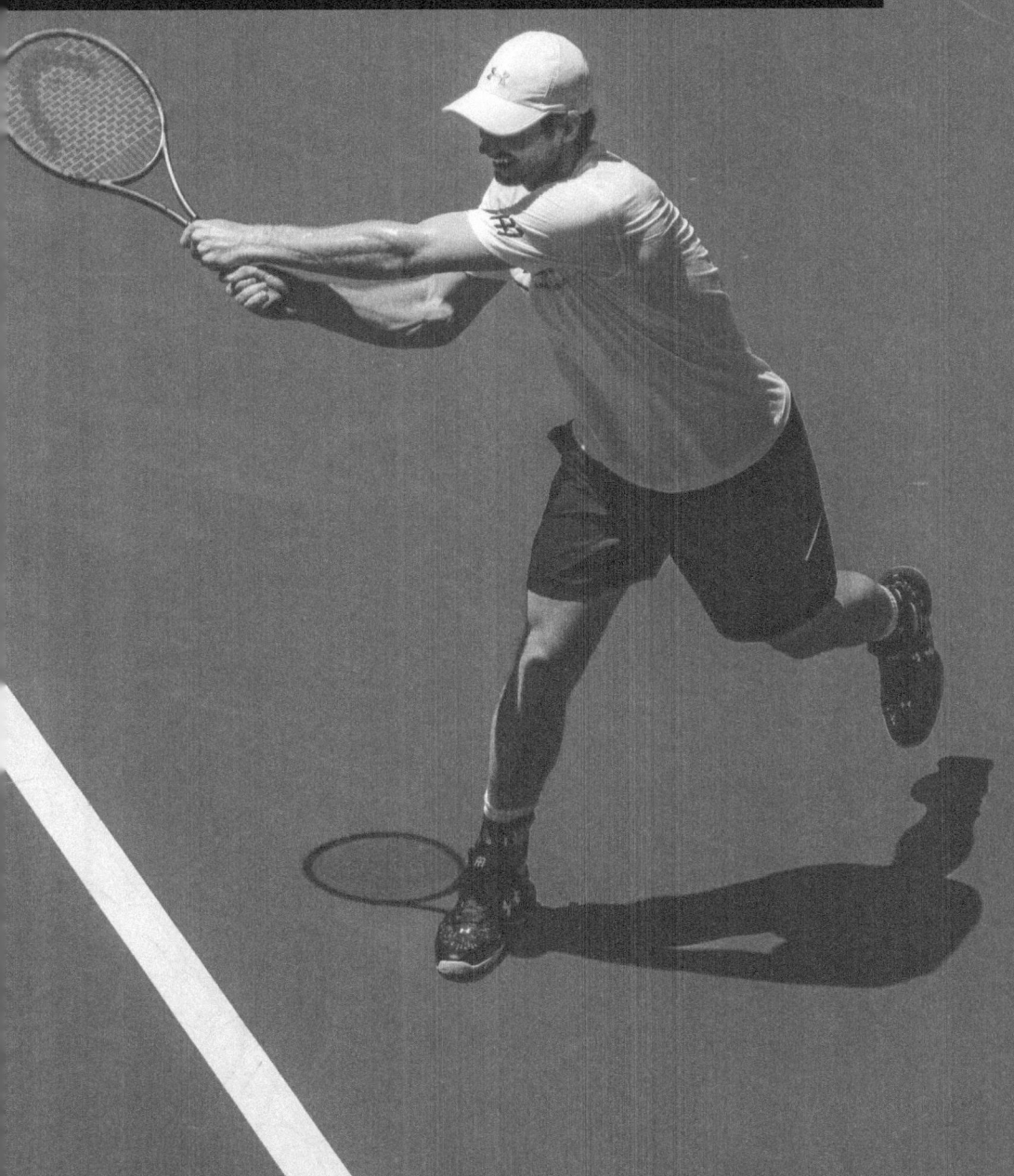

CBD Isolate vs. Full-Spectrum Hemp Oil

Why Is Full-Spectrum Better?

WHILE the most commonly known phytocannabinoid, CBD, offers great benefits on its own, it's more potent when it's extracted along with all of the other compounds contained in the hemp plant. The most significant synergy comes from an extract containing the full spectrum of phytocannabinoids (including CBD) that are contained within hemp oil.

"Full-spectrum" refers to oil extracted from the hemp plant without isolating specific compounds, which means that the oil contains a far broader range of nutrient properties than what exists when CBD is artificially isolated and concentrated after being extracted from hemp oil, as it is in many products currently on the market. Full-spectrum hemp oil harnesses the plant's real power, its complete phytocannabinoid profile, while artificially isolated CBD extracts do not.

The science now shows that the full spectrum of phytocannabinoids in hemp oil can best fine-tune the body's internal endocannabinoid system. The phytocannabinoids contained within full-spectrum hemp oil work synergistically with one another within the system, and the system runs optimally, not like a violin solo, but like a symphony performance, in which all of the instruments play a role.

Studies now show that the most powerful benefits come when all of the phytocannabinoids in full-spectrum hemp oil work together in harmony. The hand-in-hand work between all of the phytocannabinoids and the cannabinoid receptors is one type of interaction commonly referred to as the "entourage effect," conveying the idea that cannabinoids work most effectively when they dance in harmony, as a group, rather than when they are isolated.

A 2015 study by the Lautenberg Center for General Tumor Immunology in Jerusalem,[15] for example, endorsed the power of the entourage effect inherent in full-spectrum oil extract. Mice receiving high doses of CBD from full-spectrum hemp oil experienced greater relief than those subjected to the same doses of CBD isolate.

26 PLANTS, PERFORMANCE AND THE ENDOCANNABINOID SYSTEM

The full power of CBD is only realized when it is part of a symphony, which is why full-spectrum hemp oil is so vital.* And the range of instruments does not stop with phytocannabinoids—in the past few years, scientists have discovered that a wide variety of plants interact with the ECS in ways that contribute to the music's beautiful melodies and resonance. The best health and performance wellness strategies deploy as many of these instruments as possible.

---

* Nonetheless, for ease of reading going forward, when we refer to CBD in the remaining pages we mean it to include all of the cannabinoids derived from full-spectrum hemp extract.

5 PHYTOCANNABINOIDS FOR POTENT ENERGY AND ENDURANCE

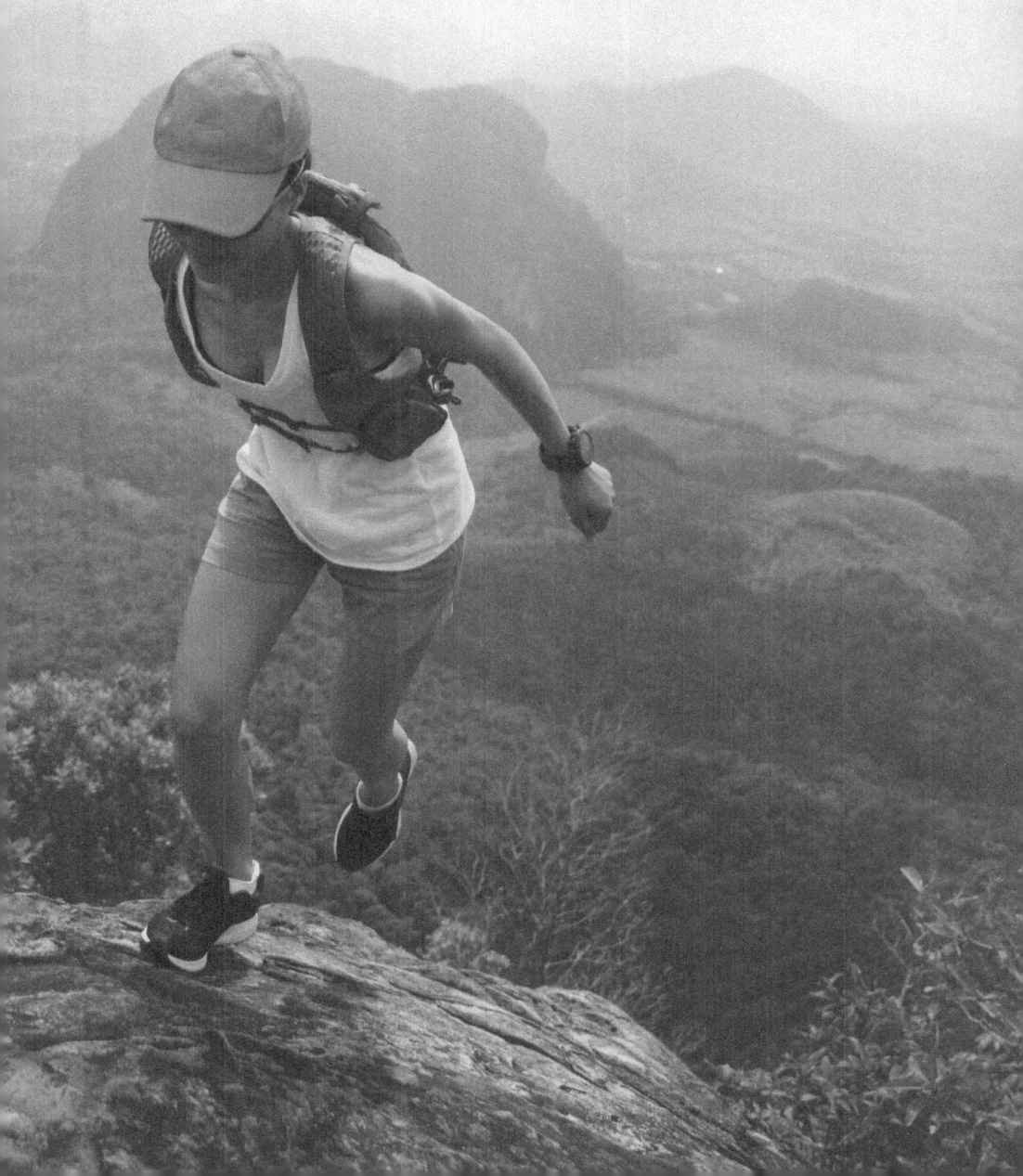

Phytocannabinoids for Potent Energy and Endurance

ENERGY bars. Espresso shots. Bagels. Ginseng shooters. When it comes to training and competition, few things are more important to athletes than energy, and they rely upon a wide range of substances for juice injections. Most of the energy gambits are one-dimensional—like carbohydrate-packed bagels, they provide quick bursts of fuel, or like espresso shots, they amp energy for short periods of time, with all the hallmarks of stimulants: racing mind, heart palpitations, and sweats.

Boosting Energy at the Cellular Level

Phytocannabinoids boost energy through entirely different means. Instead of flooding the body with stimulants, which are substances that are not naturally found within the body, phytocannabinoids work with the endocannabinoid system to improve energy in ways that fit with the body's natural rhythms. Again, we return to homeostasis and the analogy of body's machinery: rather than overloading the engine with foreign substances (which can tax the body's harmony and certainly reduce its chances of achieving a balanced hum), phytocannabinoids like CBD optimize the body's own abilities to generate high levels of energy for peak performance.

One of CBD's energy-raising triumphs hinges on CBD's positive impacts on the body's mitochondria, which serve as *the* power plant for cells[16] and hence energy production throughout the brain and body. CBD helps keep mitochondria active, which strengthens them—and mitochondria are essential partners in regulating the body's energy. Among other things, mitochondria use what is called the Krebs Cycle chemical reaction[17] to convert food to energy. Stronger mitochondria (thank you, CBD) lead to enhanced energy.

Also, CBD activates serotonin receptors in the brain,[18] and serotonin levels are related to energy. Higher levels of serotonin often lead to a more positive outlook on life and increased energy, while low serotonin levels are tied to depression and lethargy. Research by both the University of São Paulo in Brazil[19] and King's College in London[20] show that CBD helps interfere with a complex series of processes that slow down or even stop serotonin production. By blocking naturally occurring genetic glitches that depress serotonin levels, CBD in effect ensures that serotonin levels remain where they should be—in harmony with the rest of the body, for optimum contentment and robust energy.

CBD helps keep mitochondria active, which strengthens them—and mitochondria are essential partners in regulating the body's energy.

Enhancing Endurance

The most accomplished athletes grapple with endurance every day—for most of them, the scale of their triumphs relates directly to how well they soldier on through the roadblocks set before them. Much of the struggle happens in the brain rather than the biceps. Those able

Phytocannabinoids' ability to invoke and prolong the runner's high is extremely beneficial for many athletes who are training hard for long periods of time.

to transform nagging pain and difficulty into pleasure, or at least some state of contentment, tend to reach the highest levels of athletic achievement. Among endurance runners, the pleasure-through-pain feeling that emerges is called the "runner's high."[21]

Recent research shows that the endocannabinoid system contains two primary endocannabinoids (again, endocannabinoids are the body's own homegrown type of cannabinoid), and one of them, anandamide,[22] appears to be instrumental in the blossoming of runner's high—in fact, anandamide is referred to as the "bliss molecule," its name derived from the Sanskrit word for bliss, *ananda*. The phytocannabinoid connection? Phytocannabinoids communicate with anandamide[23] in such a way that the blissful feeling is expressed by the body with more ease. The science is complex, but to summarize, phytocannabinoids, particularly CBD, help increase levels of anandamide so that those blissful feelings are more easily conjured, lengthened, and stabilized.

Bliss rocks, especially for athletes trudging up mountain trails or dipping into that seventy-fifth minute on the soccer field. But recent research shows that reaching that exercise-induced state of bliss comes more naturally to some than to others. Richard Friedman, a professor of clinical psychiatry at Weill Cornell Medical College, studies anandamide closely, and in an editorial for the New York Times[24] wrote, "For the first time, scientists have demonstrated that a genetic variation in the brain makes some people inherently less anxious, and more able to forget fearful and unpleasant experiences. This lucky genetic mutation produces higher levels of anandamide—the so-called bliss molecule and our own natural marijuana—in our brains."

CBD doesn't deliver a one-dimensional, single-shot stimulant that briefly thrusts the body into overdrive before fading away. Instead, it helps the body remain vigorous and resilient throughout the duration of athletic pursuits.

For those blessed with the genetic quirk, bliss (and thus, greater endurance) during exercise is achieved with greater ease. Meanwhile, some people suffer from genetics that diminish anandamide production, a condition that researchers have tied to depression, among other things.

Why does this matter to athletes? Phytocannabinoids' ability to invoke and prolong the runner's high is extremely beneficial for many athletes who are training hard for long periods of time. The "runner's high" feeling is gold for endurance: instead of fixing on the negatives (pain, boredom) those savoring runner's high can sink into pleasure instead. So anything that strengthens that natural condition, such as CBD, is a bonus.

When phytocannabinoids like CBD are incorporated into daily life, heightened and sustained energy levels provide a helping hand throughout the day while at the same time delivering longer-term endurance sufficient to meet the challenges imposed upon the body in training and competition. CBD doesn't deliver a one-dimensional, single-shot stimulant that briefly thrusts the body into overdrive before fading away. Instead, it helps the body remain vigorous and resilient for the duration of athletic pursuits.

6 CBD FOR STRESS-BUSTING AND ANXIETY REDUCTION

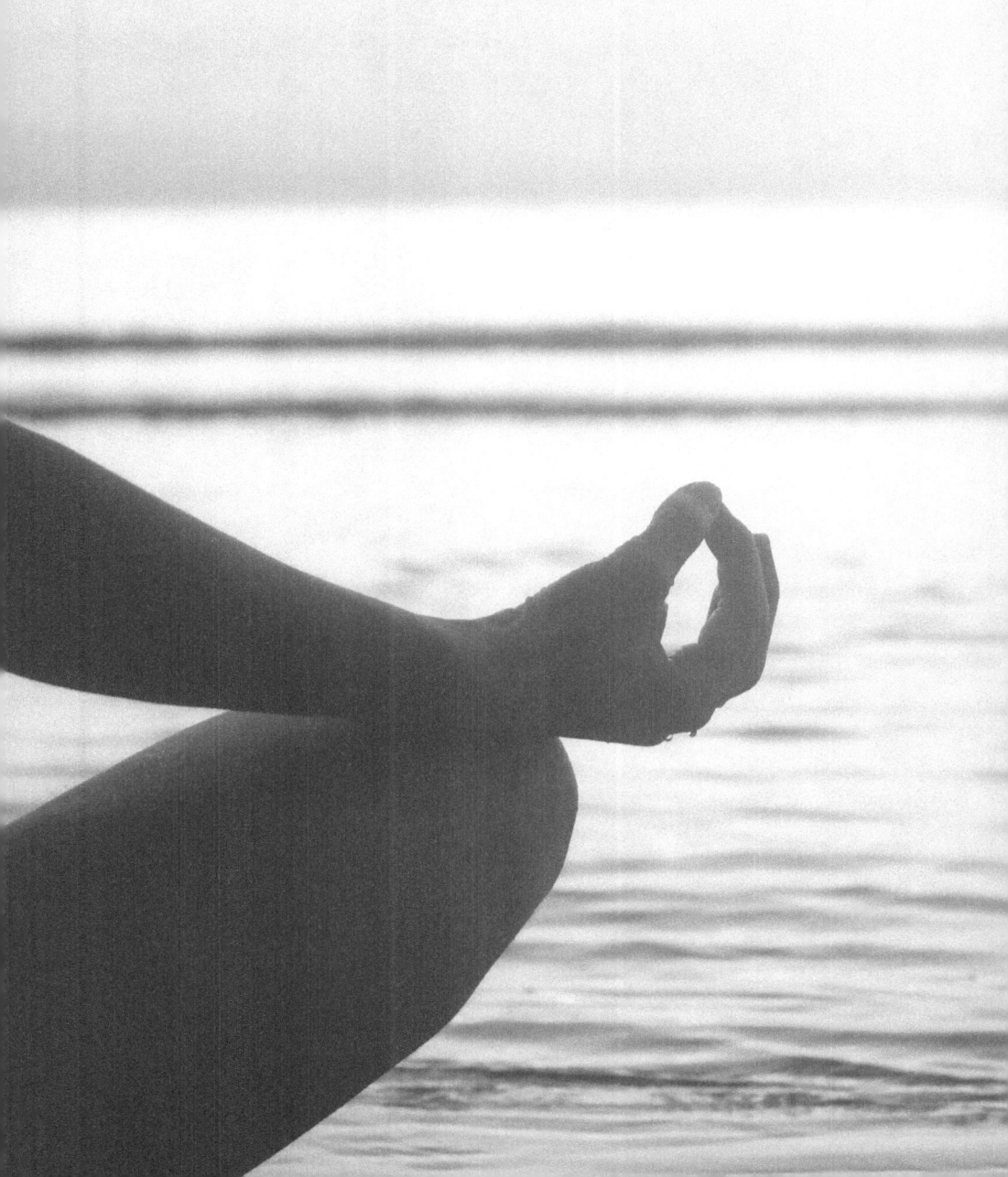

CBD for Stress-Busting and Anxiety Reduction

STRESS come at athletes from all sides—the normal stress they confront in their daily lives (shuttling kids around during busy days, work demands, health worries, etc.) along with both the physical and mental stress that training and competing invite. Bodies grow exhausted, and become less efficient at handling the daily parade of pressures. Sickness and burnout go hand in hand, due to the body's inability to handle stress. Brains, drained of vigor, lose their edge; mental keenness dulls and performance nosedives.

This is where CBD comes in. It's an anxiety-buster.[25] Anxiety, which is a reaction to stress, leads to a wide variety of health conditions, including a weakened immune system, an overworked nervous system, weaker respiratory functions, cardiovascular problems, and stomach and digestive tract issues. All of these interfere with the athlete's journey, and CBD's role in managing anxiety is yet another boon for athletes. It's all (well, at least mostly) about serotonin. Recent studies show CBD elevates serotonin levels in the brain.

Many pharmaceutical antidepressants are called selective serotonin reuptake inhibitors (SSRIs),[26] which work, in effect, to provide the body more access to serotonin. Serotonin is vital for mood health, and by helping to improve mood, serotonin serves as an important tool for muzzling anxiety (and managing stress). Research from Spain[27] found that CBD may be more effective than even SSRIs in improving the way serotonin interacts with the brain. The science is complicated, but in effect, research shows that CBD might help block processes that diminish serotonin in the brain, thereby leading to improved brain access to serotonin. And as we mentioned earlier, increased serotonin is tied to decreased anxiety and hence more resourcefulness in coping with stress.

Further clinical research buttresses the idea that CBD fights anxiety.[28] One study in Brazil[29] showed that study participants who took

CBD reported reduced anxiety levels, and follow-up brain scans confirmed the participants' subjective testimonials. Another Brazilian study[30] monitored people who suffered from Social Anxiety Disorder during a public speaking test. Researchers found participants in the study who consumed CBD experienced "significantly reduced anxiety," while the placebo group suffered from higher anxiety.

CBD may be more effective than even SSRIs in improving the way serotonin interacts with the brain.

CBD's role in serotonin management is key to understanding how the cannabinoid muffles anxiety and flattens stress. But CBD's stress-battling arsenal extends beyond serotonin.

Phytocannabinoids like CBD may protect against excess stress by reducing recurring activation of the hypothalamus-pituitary-adrenal (HPA) axis, which is the cause of much of the chronic stress experienced in modern life.

Another study, this one from Spain, found that CBD may help the hippocampus to regenerate neurons[31] —an important finding, because the hippocampus[32] is central to brain activity. Research reveals that people suffering from anxiety and depression exhibit a relatively small hippocampus, and successful treatment of depression can lead to fresh neurons in the hippocampus, as well as a larger hippocampus. The connection between the hippocampus, anxiety, and CBD looks promising. By buttressing the hippocampus, CBD can help fight anxiety—including anxious feelings stemming from stress.

CBD also directly impacts our response to and ability to manage stress through its influence on the endocrine system, which consists of glands throughout the body that regulate everything from metabolism and energy to sex drive. Science indicates that phytocannabinoids like CBD may protect against excess stress by reducing recurring activation of the hypothalamus-pituitary-adrenal (HPA) axis, which is the cause of much of the chronic stress experienced in modern life.[33]

Additionally, studies show that CBD significantly reduces cortisol levels,[34] which repeatedly spike when the HPA axis is overly active and are responsible for the harmful effects of chronic stress, including the negative impacts that cortisol has on deep, restful sleep.[35]

7 CBD FOR DEEP SLEEP

CBD For Deep Sleep

WHAT does sleep have to do with athletics? Let's return to the engine metaphor. While the engine is pumping especially hard during exercise, those "mechanics" in the endocannabinoid system are busy adjusting belts, adding oil, and efficiently getting fuel to the right places. But like any engine, the body's cannot run at full throttle forever. Without downtime, things begin to break down: joints and muscles ache and sometimes even experience sharp pain, the mind grows foggy, fuel gets exhausted, and the willpower essential for training and competing drains away. At this point, the body craves just sitting, some stretching, lots of water and fresh fuel. But it is only during sound sleep that true replenishment and restoration takes place. For athletes, solid sleep is as essential as fuel and strength. And the same goes for everybody soldiering through life's struggles—without solid sleep, problems tend to build upon one another and escalate until everything comes crashing down.

The importance of sleep is another reason athletes increasingly are turning to CBD. Phytocannabinoids help the body drift into extremely restorative states of rest,[36] without the nasty side-effects that often come with prescription, over-the-counter, and herbal sedatives.

Anxiety serves as a principal sleep inhibitor, and CBD research shows that the compound is capable of reducing anxiety—a key step in improving sleep quality (see more on anxiety and CBD in chapter six, **CBD For Stress-Busting**). Pain is another sleep impediment (if not destroyer), and CBD research demonstrates that the cannabinoid reduces chronic pain (read more about connections between CBD and pain management in the next chapter, **CBD For Beating Inflammation**).

The diminished anxiety and pain that CBD promotes also supports deeper sleep patterns. But CBD's help with sleep doesn't stop there. Studies show that CBD may help prolong the third stage of non-REM sleep,[37] which researchers believe improves overall sleep quality. The REM (rapid eye movement) portions of a night of sleep represent the most active (and least restful) part of the under-the-covers session—

this is when most intense dreaming occurs. While REM sleep is important, so too is non-REM sleep, and people suffering from different sleep issues often experience prolonged bouts of REM. Research suggesting that CBD prolongs non-REM sleep holds further promise for CBD as a sleep aid.

The CBD approach—minimizing sleep-busters like anxiety and pain, and diminishing REM sleep—is much better than the sedative route: landing a knockout punch. While sedatives often do work, the sleep usually comes at a steep price: morning grogginess. In addition, the knockout doesn't always persist for everybody. People pop the sedative, fall asleep easily, but wake up four to six hours later because the pill has stopped working, so the grogginess is exacerbated: they feel cloudy from the sedative, but since they didn't fall into a long, restful sleep, the clouds thicken into a gray mantle of gloom.

As the medical and scientific community begins to engage more routinely with the hemp plant, more and more research emerges detailing the plant's manifold wellness compounds and potential uses.

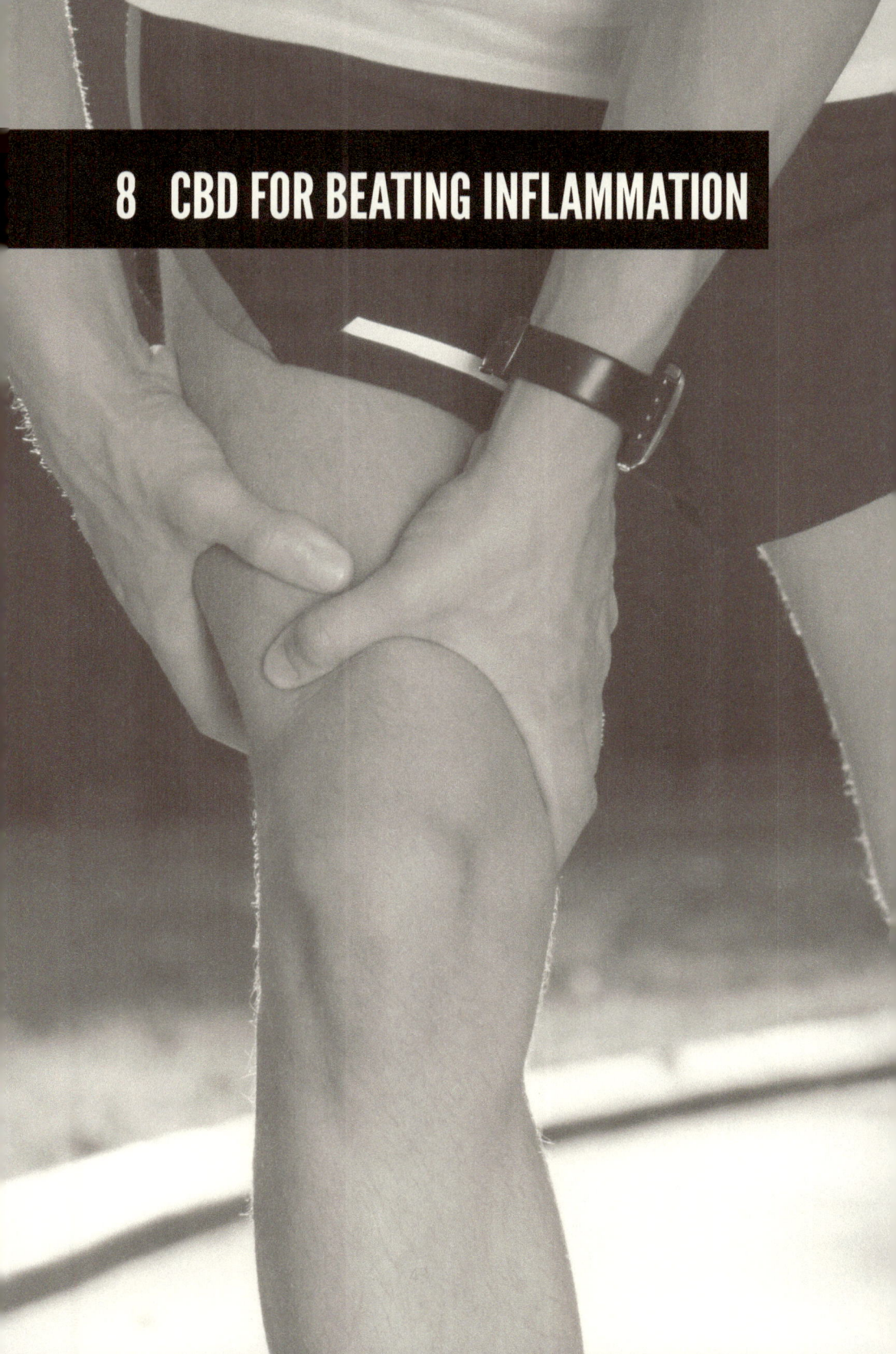

8 CBD FOR BEATING INFLAMMATION

CBD for Beating Inflammation

THE THROBBING KNEE after a long run. The radiating pain from the rotator cuff following an intense day of climbing. The fire in the hip after an afternoon of skinning up slopes and then tearing down them. What is that torment? In many cases, it's inflammation. And inflammation is yet another sphere of human health where CBD plays an important role.[38]

Over the past five years, the subject of inflammation has moved into the center of the national health zeitgeist. Trends like the gluten-free and paleo diets find their roots in concerns about inflammation. Among the world's panoply of diseases, inflammation gets singled out as a very, *very* big part of the problem. Seven out of the ten leading causes of mortality are tied to inflammation, including heart disease, cancer, stroke, and diabetes. And among athletes, of course, inflammation is simply part of daily life—post-training regimens always hinge at least in part upon strategies for mitigating that meddlesome inflammation.

Numerous studies from around the world now indicate CBD's role in reducing pain and inflammation related to acute and chronic conditions like arthritis. The intersection of CBD and inflammation is now a subject of intense study, and its use among athletes to reduce inflammation and pain has made headlines in recent years.

The science behind CBD's effectiveness in managing inflammation includes an important cannabinoid "receptor" in the nervous system, called CB2.[39] Before CBD fully enters the nervous system and works with the body for different effects, CB2 interacts with it—and CBD stimulates the CB2 receptors. Good news: CB2 is deeply involved with the body's immune system, which helps mitigate the ill effects of inflammation.

This relationship between CB2 and CBD informs some of the good news coming out of different scientific studies. One study, from researchers at Imperial College London, showed that CBD reduced inflammation in mice by fifty percent.[40] Another study by G.W. Pharmaceuticals[41] showed promise in treating rheumatoid arthritis, a disease characterized by crippling body-wide inflammation. More? A University of Kentucky study[42] in 2016 found that CBD reduced inflammation and pain in arthritic rats. Researchers at the National Institute of Health conducted a study showing that inflammatory and neuropathic pain can be effectively treated with CBD.[43]

Based on these emerging studies about CBD's impact on acute and chronic inflammation, it appears that CBD may be more powerful than many of the most commonly recommended natural products for inflammation like Vitamin C, fish oil, turmeric and resveratrol. Combining CBD with these natural ingredients may have an even greater impact.

And it's not just scientists experimenting with CBD to explore its inflammation-fighting properties. Athletes from a wide range of sports, including professional football, have publicly endorsed CBD's ability to help them manage often crippling inflammation and pain.

"I was open for anything," former Denver Broncos quarterback Jake Plummer told CBS News.[44] "And once I tried it and was consistent on CBD, that's when I realized, 'Wow, this stuff works.'"

Plummer and numerous other professional football players have become CBD ambassadors, evangelizing about the power of the cannabinoid to manage pain and inflammation and extolling it over opiates and analgesics.

But the NFL continues to ban CBD for players currently suiting up. Since CBD is derived from hemp, and the hemp plant is related to cannabis, the League has lumped together everything related to hemp, even though hemp products have no psychoactive effect.

Is CBD Addictive or Unsafe?

While the NFL and other professional sports associations in the U.S. continue to ban CBD, other international organizations are more enlightened. In September of 2017, the World Anti-Doping Agency (WADA) removed CBD from its 2018 list of prohibited substances.[45] The move will please athletes like UFC star fighter Nate Diaz, who made waves in 2016 when he publicly took draws from a vape pen filled with CBD after a fight.[46] "It's CBD," he said. "It helps with the healing process and inflammation, stuff like that."

Additionally, since WADA rules govern Olympic athletes, Olympic athletes will be able to use CBD starting in 2018.[47] This is a landmark decision that will likely send ripples through professional athletics worldwide.

Finally, in late 2017, a report[48] from the World Health Organization (WHO)[49] found there is no evidence that CBD presents any public health concerns, nor is it addictive, and that it should not be regulated as a controlled substance. The WHO report also highlighted that there is "preliminary evidence" CBD could be useful in treating Alzheimer's disease,[50] cancer, psychosis, Parkinson's disease, and other serious conditions.[51]

9 THE CBD ADVANTAGE FOR ATHLETES

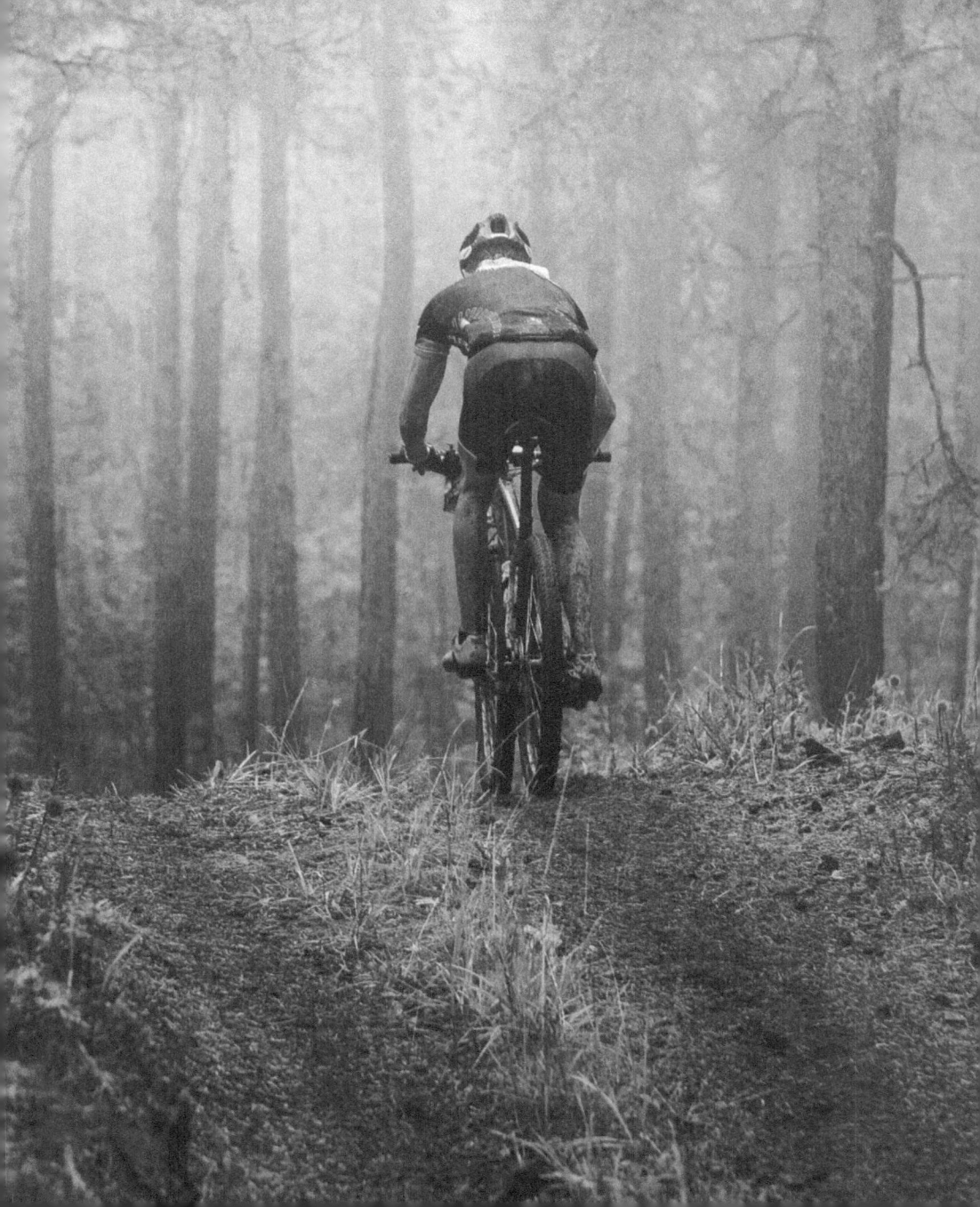

The CBD Advantage for Athletes

An Unmatched Edge

AS PHYTOCANNABINOIDS like CBD receive increasing clinical scrutiny, the body of research illustrating the hemp plant's bounty of wellness benefits and applications blossoms. At the same time, strong word-of-mouth between athletes has turned many on to the power of hemp and CBD.

Soothed inflammation and pain. Deep sleep. Diminished, if not vanquished, anxiety and stress. Enriched and heightened energy. These serve as the foundations of athletic performance, and CBD attends to them all by bolstering the body's own reserves of health-nurturing power rather than merely filling the body with external substances delivering short-term effects. Given the wide spectrum of ways hemp supports performance and recovery, it appears to be the adaptogen of all adaptogens—an unparalleled uber-adaptogen. Our bodies are miracles, filled with all that most of us need to thrive while running up mountains, snowboarding down couloirs, or shooting hoops. But most bodies need help to get all of the cylinders firing at maximum capacity, to make sure those pistons keep pumping hard, and to help coordinate all of the body's moving parts in such a way that everything hums. And CBD, unlike any other supplement in history, helps the body make its beautiful music.

10 BEYOND CBD

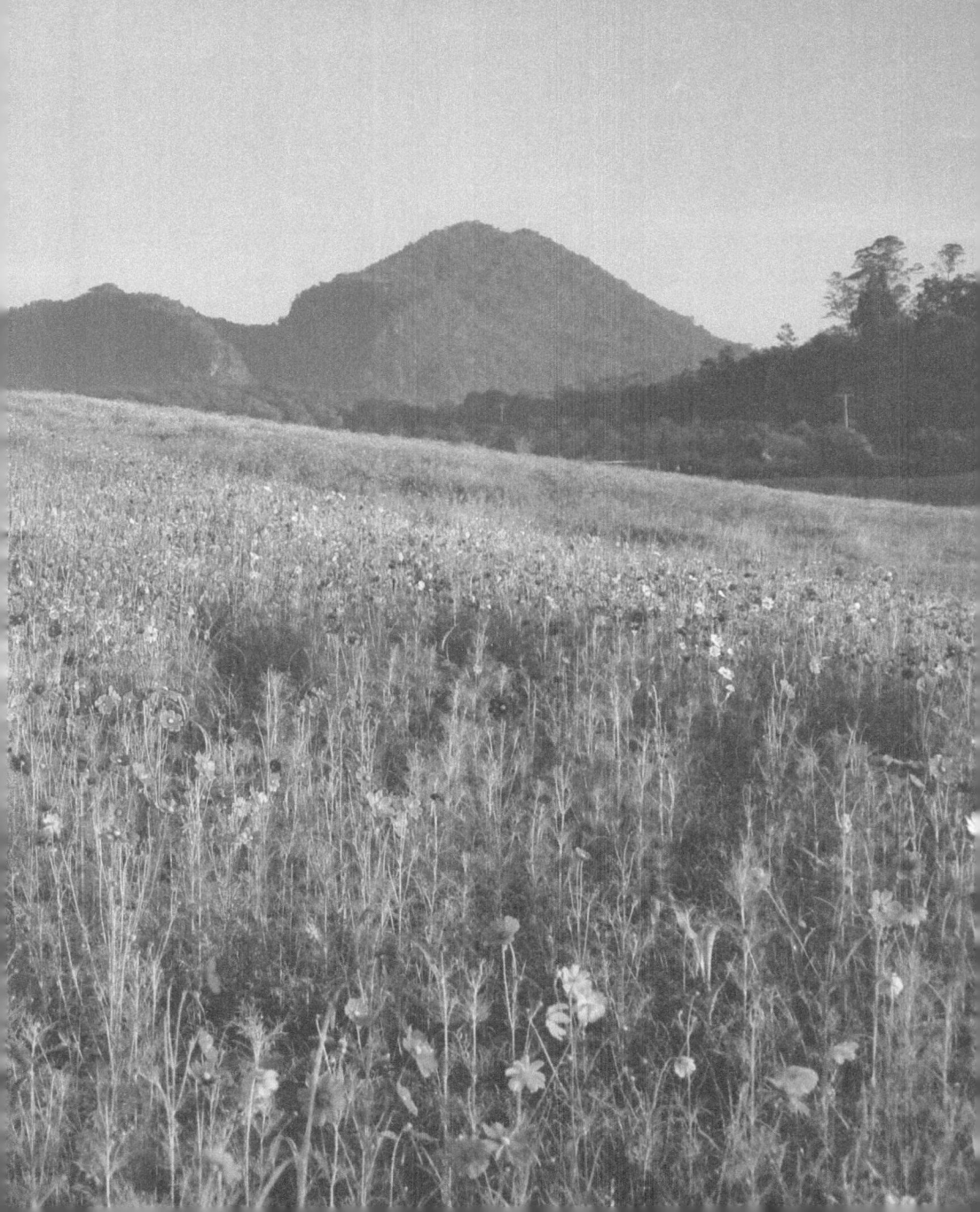

Beyond CBD

The Performance Boost of other Powerhouse Plants

LEARNING how to incorporate CBD into any high-stress lifestyle—from professional athlete to professional parent—offers immense benefits that we've described in this book: the potential for enhanced sleep, boosted endurance, optimized recovery, managed stress and anxiety, and ramped-up energy.

But CBD's advantages can grow even more profound with the addition of other plant and mineral extracts. Research is now showing that other plants also contain compounds that feed the endocannabinoid system,[52] including ginger, magnolia, and boswellia. In addition, numerous other plants have been studied extensively for their health-promoting properties, which appear to be magnified when combined with hemp.

Boswellia,[53] an herbal extract derived from an Indian tree, has been shown to mitigate muscle and joint inflammation, also without the side-effects that come from analgesics like ibuprofen. Tart cherry, too, has been shown to support normal inflammatory response.[54] Bromelain,[55] papain,[56] and serrepeptase[57] are a trio of enzymes that actually *support* inflammation. Our muscles and joints become inflamed for a reason (the process leads to recovery); by effectively clearing out the debris scattered throughout muscles and joints, these enzymes help the body work efficiently through the inflammation process and lead it to faster and more complete recovery. Cordyceps,[58] a kind of fungus, is used to fight free radicals and boost endurance. Jamaica dogwood[59] and white willow bark help soothe the discomfort associated with overstimulated nerve endings.

The amino acid referred to as GABA is leveraged to calm the central nervous system and help reduce insomnia.[60] 5-HTP, a chemical by-product of the protein building block L-tryptophan, supports neurotransmitters and can lead to diminished anxiety and improved sleep.[61] California poppy,[62] magnolia bark,[63] and skullcap[64] are all deeply restorative botanicals. Many plant extracts aid with energy expansion and maintenance, including rhodiola,[65] schisandra,[66] citrus aurantium,[67] green tea extract,[68] ashwagandha,[69] and more.

For all botanicals, health goals are only achieved when they are fully absorbed into the body. And absorption can be an issue with certain kinds of botanicals in supplement form, including hemp. But plants like ginger that improve digestion are key partners in the ongoing quest to optimize absorption, as well as the curcuminoids found in turmeric. By combining curcuminoids with hemp extract, evidence indicates that the nutrients in the hemp may be more effectively absorbed in the body.

Meanwhile, organs like the liver are constantly under assault, and stressful athletic and life pursuits can tax the liver. So plants like milk thistle,[70] which target liver health, are welcome.

Different health needs, such as sleep, energy, and recovery, demand diverse combinations of botanicals. Somebody seeking sleep, for example, would not turn to an adaptogen like ginseng, nor would an athlete about to head out on a trail run reach for chamomile, a flower well-known for its calming and restorative effects.

The best plant-based strategies for achieving and maintaining optimal wellness and performance turn to combinations of complementary botanicals—everything from hemp oil extract to Vitamin B12 and ginger root extract.

Plant Power Case Studies

NFL Lineman Kyle Turley's Painful Journey, and the CBD Solution

After eight seasons as an NFL offensive lineman for the New Orleans Saints, St. Louis Rams, and Kansas City Chiefs, Kyle Turley's battered body ached. Plates and screws decorated different body parts. Bone-on-bone arthritis turned motions most people take for granted into adventures in pain. Neuropathy in his feet produced chronic pain that affected everything from walking to sleeping.

Doctors prescribed opiates, muscle relaxers, sleep aids, drugs to deal with neurological issues. "I deal with unbelievable pain and aches that would disable most people, forcing them to be stuck at home. And that was happening to me," he said.

Then he discovered CBD,[71] and it changed his life. Physical pain, mental struggles, emotional challenges—for Turley, CBD was instrumental in managing the aftermath of his grueling NFL career.

Now living in California, where he grew up, Turley is active in Athletes for Care, a nonprofit that aims not only to upend stigmas associated with the cannabis plant, including the phytocannabinoid CBD derived from hemp, but to evangelize on behalf of the plant's myriad powers. We talked with Turley about his experiences with CBD, and the role he thinks CBD can play for athletes.

After the NFL, like a lot of players, you wrestled with a host of medical issues, and doctors became a big part of your life. Much of their help came in the form of prescription drugs. Why did you seek other solutions to your health challenges?

TURLEY: Painkillers don't kill pain; they mask it. When you realize these things aren't really working, that they are not giving you your life back, it's a simple choice. You encounter cannabinoids and learn that they deal with your endocannabinoid system, that they help direct relief to your body naturally. The pharmaceuticals have consequences. The side effects are real. They paint these pretty pictures in the commercials, but they list the side effects too. And again—they are real.

Shortly after you found CBD, you became a prominent champion for the cannabinoid. Why?

TURLEY: CBD is a life changer. Having CBD has been a night and day shift in how I deal with everything. It really works with anxiety and stress, and not just for recovering athletes like me. Wide receivers today who use CBD notice they are not having missteps. They focus on the ball without anxiety and stress, and they are their best selves at that moment. That's how I think about CBD. It doesn't make you better. It makes you your best you.

Do you think CBD will be an important sports supplement?

TURLEY: With CBD you are focused. Ready. You don't let distractions interfere with your performance. When your mind is in focus as an athlete, your performance level will be increased. And with CBD we aren't really talking about introducing something foreign to the body. We are talking about igniting the endocannabinoid system, and CBD alone can do that. It has an unbelievable power to be a sports supplement. It deals with inflammation. It deals with issues that come with competing, including performing and essentially being on stage.

Do you see CBD being more widely embraced among athletes?

TURLEY: It's a tidal wave. It has grown exponentially. Every sport, at every level, is engaged with this. Pro surfers. NFL players and owners. In sports you have injuries—it's inherent. We have had enough experience with pharmaceuticals. We are in dire need of better solutions and I don't think there is anything else out there right now more effective than CBD.

Endurance Trail Runner Avery Collins's CBD Breakthrough

He runs long—as much as a hundred miles. And ultramarathoner Avery Collins[72] does this over and over again, competing (and routinely finishing as a race leader) in grueling ultramarathons like the Western States 100,[73] the Grindstone 100,[74] the Georgia Death Race,[75] and more.

Hard training gets the credit for so much success at such an early age (he began winning competitions in his early twenties). But Collins champions something else, too, for his parade of endurance triumphs: phytocannabinoids, including CBD. "Several years ago, after my finish at the Indiana Trail 100,[76] I developed a golf-ball sized injury in my Achilles," Collins told Ultimate Guide. "It was a problem, even more so because I was competing in another hundred-mile ultra just seventeen days later."

Collins slathered cream on his screaming Achilles—cream infused with CBD. And less than two weeks later, the brutal injury vanished. "I don't know what happened, but the inflammation just disappeared and I felt like there was far more blood flow in the injured area," says Collins. "The bottom line is I started running almost immediately and it allowed me to complete my next race."

Since then, Collins has used CBD as a regular training partner. It eases inflammation—a persistent and often training-ending condition for endurance athletes—and dulls pain. Injuries recede more swiftly. And Collins believes CBD helps diminish anxiety and stress, which in the past led to digestion problems and stomach pain. All of these CBD advantages get him back out on his Steamboat Springs, Colorado trails more quickly than prior to his embrace of CBD.

Running long races represents Collins' career and life; training is a daily activity, and tough competitions constantly loom before him. Enriching his training regimen with CBD fortifies his focus and drive, alleviates the inevitable aches, pains, and injuries, and helps him soldier through the many athletic challenges he confronts every day.

And he is not alone. Endurance athletes around the world are finding relief and renewed vigor through the use of cannabinoids like

CBD.[77] So many professional and ambitious athletes are turning to CBD, from UFC fighters bloodying each other in the ring to ultra-marathoners speeding up and down steep mountain trails, that the natural compound is becoming as essential to athletes as energy bars and electrolyte-infused water.

But there is a big difference. The other training tools are just along for the training or competition ride. But CBD and other plant-based extracts are there to enhance not only performance but life overall.

Conclusion

I HOPE you now have much of the information and many of the answers you wanted when you purchased this book. Importantly, we continue to follow the latest studies, research and athlete case studies that speak to the power of hemp and the other plants highlighted in the book. If you would like updates on our research, or you have a case study to share for a future edition of this book, you can do so here: www.plantsforperformance.com/follow.

Finally, we want to say thank you for purchasing this book and allowing us the opportunity to share our developing knowledge and experience with you. We hope this book enables you to better understand and explore for yourself the benefits of hemp and these other performance plants. Most importantly, we hope it provided you with some information and inspiration to conquer greater and greater feats in your life.

Learn About the Authors

Don McLaughlin

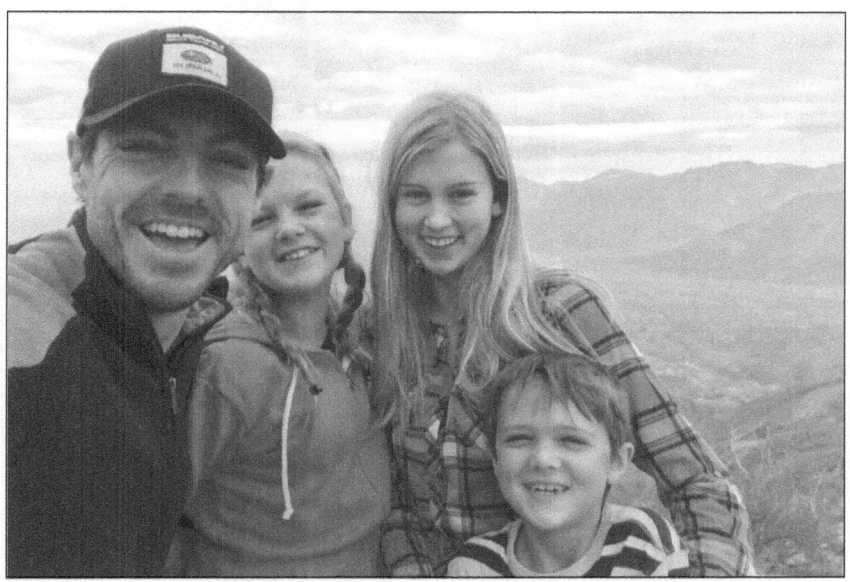

Don is a father of three, author, wellness advocate, and ultra endurance athlete. A former trial lawyer of nearly twenty years, Don's legal career included service as an assistant district attorney, litigator at a prominent Colorado law firm, and in-house corporate lawyer at a Fortune 500. As a corporate lawyer, Don became a nationally recognized expert in the areas of electronic data retrieval, analysis, and management. Subsequently Don founded and served as CEO of Falcon Discovery, a legal consulting and tech services firm serving the Fortune 500. As CEO of a rapidly growing, multi-million dollar firm that handled some of the highest profile legal cases in the country, he faced intense stress and high pressure 24/7. Following years of prolonged burnout, Don finally hit bottom in 2012. After what he can only describe as divine intervention, Don became inspired to overhaul his diet and begin running long-distance, ultra endurance trail races in the Colorado Rockies. He incorporated hemp and other plant extracts into a new health regime, and developed a series of wellness practices to advance his recovery and sustain high performance. With these changes, nearly everything in his life turned around, and Don's business and personal life flourished. Within months his running distances doubled and tripled, and the business grew like never before. He subsequently sold Falcon Discovery and stepped down in 2017 to support and inspire others with the lessons that he learned. To this end Don is finishing work on his first book, which will be published in early 2019. Additionally,

Don recently founded PurePower, a health and wellness company dedicated to tapping into the transformative power of hemp and other powerful plants, and a set of high-performance practices he calls Inside-Out Performance. Don lives outside Steamboat Springs, Colorado with his three children, several horses, and his trail-running champion rescue dog, Sophie. For more information, go to www.livepurepower.com or visit www.donmclaughlinjr.com.

Doug Brown

Douglas Brown spent more than 20 years as a journalist, covering everything from the White House and Capitol Hill to crime in New Mexico to technology, food, and wine. Now he is a founding partner at Campfire Content, a content agency with offices in Boulder and Vail, Colorado. Doug began experimenting with CBD in 2017, as his trail running grew more ambitious, and now he is a CBD champion. Doug lives in Boulder with Annie Brown and their two daughters, Stella and Ruby.

Notes

Chapter One: A Ski Pro's Story

1. Jakob Schiller, "The Ski Industry's 6 Most Charismatic Icons," *Outside Online*, February 3, 2016, https://www.outsideonline.com/2053226/ski-industrys-6-most-charismatic-icons.

2. Dynafit, *From the Road*, YouTube, https://www.youtube.com/watch?v=-zKXIJnv8_4.

3. "What Is CBD? Definition of Cannabidiol & CBD Oil," Project CBD, https://www.projectcbd.org/about/what-is-cbd.

4. Jim McAlpine bio, SXSW 2017 Schedule, https://schedule.sxsw.com/2017/speakers/3443.

5. 420 Games website, https://420games.civilized.life. (As of February 13, 2019, this is a "coming soon" web page.)

6. "Athletes for CARE website, https://www.athletesforcare.org.

Chapter Two: Hemp as Uber Adaptogen

7. Perry Solomon, "Marijuana, Cannabinoids and Homeostasis: A Balancing Act," *HelloMD*, https://www.hellomd.com/health-wellness/56b27573fe98a100080001f1/marijuana-cannabinoids-and-homeostasis-a-balancing-act.

Chapter Three: What is the Endocannabinoid System?

8. "The Discovery of the Endocannabinoid System and Cannabinoids," *ECHO Connection*, May 15, 2017, https://echoconnection.org/discovery-endocannabinoid-system/.

9. K. Mackie, "Cannabinoid Receptors: Where They Are and What They Do," *Journal of Neuroendocrinology* 20 Suppl 1 (May 2008): 10–14, https://www.ncbi.nlm.nih.gov/pubmed/18426493.

10 "Endocannabinoids: Overview, History, Chemical Structure," Medscape, January 26, 2018, https://emedicine.medscape.com/article/1361971-overview.

11 "Metabolic Enzymes," BPS Bioscience, https://bpsbioscience.com/metabolic-enzymes.

12 Bradley E. Alger, "Getting High on the Endocannabinoid System," *Cerebrum: The Dana Forum on Brain Science* 2013 (November 1, 2013), https://www.ncbi.nlm.nih.gov/pmc/articles/PMC3997295/.

13 Melissa Sherrard, "What Does CBD Do to Your Body?," Civilized, Oct 26, 2017, https://www.civilized.life/articles/what-cbd-does-to-body/.

14 "How Marijuana's CBD Works In The Body According To Science," Jan 22, 2019, The Fresh Toast, https://thefreshtoast.com/cannabis/how-marijuanas-cbd-works-in-the-body-according-to-science/.

Chapter Four: CBD Isolate vs. Full-Spectrum Hemp Oil

15 Ruth Gallily, Zhannah Yekhtin, and Lumír Ondřej Hanuš, "Overcoming the Bell-Shaped Dose-Response of Cannabidiol by Using Cannabis Extract Enriched in Cannabidiol," *Pharmacology & Pharmacy* 06 (February 5, 2015): 75, https://doi.org/10.4236/pp.2015.62010.

Chapter Five: Phytocannabinoids for Potent Energy and Endurance

16 Adrian Devitt-Lee, "Mitochondria Mysteries: Homeostasis, Renewal and the Endocannabinoid System," December 7, 2016, Project CBD, https://www.projectcbd.org/article/cannabinoids-and-mitochondria.

17 "Citric Acid Cycle," in Wikipedia, January 30, 2019, https://en.wikipedia.org/wiki/Citric_acid_cycle.

18 "How CBD Works," accessed February 13, 2019, https://www.projectcbd.org/how-cbd-works.

19 A. G. Sartim, F. S. Guimarães, and S. R. L. Joca, "Antidepressant-like Effect of Cannabidiol Injection into the Ventral Medial Prefrontal Cortex-Possible Involvement of 5-HT1A and CB1 Receptors," *Behavioural Brain Research* 303 (April 15, 2016): 218–27, https://doi.org/10.1016/j.bbr.2016.01.033.

20 Philip McGuire et al., "Cannabidiol (CBD) as an Adjunctive Therapy in Schizophrenia: A Multicenter Randomized Controlled Trial," *American Journal of Psychiatry* 175, no. 3 (December 15, 2017): 225–31, https://doi.org/10.1176/appi.ajp.2017.17030325.

21 Heather Hatfield, "Runner's High: Is It for Real?," WebMD, October 17, 2006, https://www.webmd.com/fitness-exercise/features/runners-high-is-it-for-real.

22 Anna Wilcox, "Anandamide (AEA): The Bliss Molecule Is the Human Version of THC," Herb, Jun 30, 2017, https://herb.co/news/health/anandamide-aea/.

23 Dale Deutsch, "Research Team Finds How CBD, a Component in Marijuana, Works Within Cells," Stony Brook Research, February 13, 2015, https://research.stonybrook.edu/news/research-team-finds-how-cbd-component-marijuana-works-within-cells.

24 Richard A. Friedman, "The Feel-Good Gene," *The New York Times*, December 21, 2017, sec. Opinion, https://www.nytimes.com/2015/03/08/opinion/sunday/the-feel-good-gene.html.

Chapter Six: CBD for Stress-Busting and Anxiety Reduction

25 "How Cannabidiol (CBD) Works for Treating Anxiety," *Leafly*, October 13, 2016, https://www.leafly.com/news/health/cbd-for-treating-anxiety.

26 "What Are SSRIs?," WebMD, accessed February 13, 2019, https://www.webmd.com/depression/ssris-myths-and-facts-about-antidepressants.

27 Leonardo BM Resstel et al., "5-HT1A Receptors Are Involved in the Cannabidiol-Induced Attenuation of Behavioural and

Cardiovascular Responses to Acute Restraint Stress in Rats," *British Journal of Pharmacology* 156, no. 1 (January 2009): 181–88, https://doi.org/10.1111/j.1476-5381.2008.00046.x.

28 David Kohn, "A Powerful New Form of Medical Marijuana, without the High," *Washington Post*, December 31, 2016, http://wapo.st/2iIRVxx?tid=ss_tw&utm_term=.6504aaef40e0.

29 Alexandre R. de Mello Schier et al., "Antidepressant-like and Anxiolytic-like Effects of Cannabidiol: A Chemical Compound of Cannabis Sativa," *CNS & Neurological Disorders Drug Targets* 13, no. 6 (2014): 953–60.

30 Mateus M Bergamaschi et al., "Cannabidiol Reduces the Anxiety Induced by Simulated Public Speaking in Treatment-Naïve Social Phobia Patients," *Neuropsychopharmacology* 36, no. 6 (May 2011): 1219–26, https://doi.org/10.1038/npp.2011.6.

31 Alline C. Campos et al., "The Anxiolytic Effect of Cannabidiol on Chronically Stressed Mice Depends on Hippocampal Neurogenesis: Involvement of the Endocannabinoid System," *The International Journal of Neuropsychopharmacology* 16, no. 6 (July 2013): 1407–19, https://doi.org/10.1017/S1461145712001502.

32 "Memory, Learning, and Emotion: The Hippocampus," PsychEducation, accessed February 13, 2019, https://psycheducation.org/brain-tours/memory-learning-and-emotion-the-hippocampus/.

33 A. W. Zuardi, F. S. Guimarães, and A. C. Moreira, "Effect of Cannabidiol on Plasma Prolactin, Growth Hormone and Cortisol in Human Volunteers," *Brazilian Journal of Medical and Biological Research = Revista Brasileira De Pesquisas Medicas E Biologicas* 26, no. 2 (February 1993): 213–17.

34 Uberto Pagotto et al., "The Emerging Role of the Endocannabinoid System in Endocrine Regulation and Energy Balance," *Endocrine Reviews* 27, no. 1 (February 1, 2006): 73–100, https://doi.org/10.1210/er.2005-0009.

35 A. W. Zuardi, F. S. Guimarães, and A. C. Moreira, "Effect of Cannabidiol on Plasma Prolactin, Growth Hormone and Cortisol in Human Volunteers," *Brazilian Journal of Medical and Biological Research = Revista Brasileira De Pesquisas Medicas E Biologicas* 26, no. 2 (February 1993): 213–17.

Chapter Seven: CBD for Deep Sleep

36 Kimberly A. Babson, James Sottile, and Danielle Morabito, "Cannabis, Cannabinoids, and Sleep: A Review of the Literature," *Current Psychiatry Reports* 19, no. 4 (March 27, 2017): 23; https://doi.org/10.1007/s11920-017-0775-9.

37 "Cannabis and Sleep: 10 Things to Know About Your Herbal Nightcap," *Leafly*, March 9, 2016, https://www.leafly.com/news/cannabis-101/cannabis-and-sleep.

Chapter Eight: CBD for Beating Inflammation

38 Studies on CBD and inflammation, accessed February 13, 2019, https://www.projectcbd.org/inflammation.

39 G. A. Cabral and L. Griffin-Thomas, "Emerging Role of the CB2 Cannabinoid Receptor in Immune Regulation and Therapeutic Prospects," *Expert Reviews in Molecular Medicine* 11 (January 20, 2009): https://doi.org/10.1017/S1462399409000957.

40 Zach Reichard, "Cannabidiol (CBD): Fighting Inflammation & Aggressive Forms of Cancer," *Medical Jane*, December 20, 2012, https://www.medicaljane.com/2012/12/20/cannabidiol-cbd-medicine-of-the-future/.

41 "Rheumatology Journal Publishes Positive Sativex® Study in Rheumatoid Arthritis," GW Pharmaceuticals, November 9, 2005, https://www.gwpharm.com/about/news/rheumatology-journal-publishes-positive-sativexr-study-rheumatoid-arthritis.

42 D.C. Hammell et al., "Transdermal Cannabidiol Reduces Inflammation and Pain-Related Behaviours in a Rat Model of

Arthritis," *European Journal of Pain* (London, England) 20, no. 6 (July 2016): 936–48, https://doi.org/10.1002/ejp.818.

43 Elizabeth J. Rahn and Andrea G. Hohmann, "Cannabinoids as Pharmacotherapies for Neuropathic Pain: From the Bench to the Bedside," *Neurotherapeutics* 6, no. 4 (October 2009): 713–37, https://doi.org/10.1016/j.nurt.2009.08.002.

44 "Could Marijuana Compound CBD Help NFL Players with Pain?," CBS News, November 30, 2016, 10:57 AM, https://www.cbsnews.com/news/nfl-marijuana-policy-push-for-cbd-marijuana-compound-cannabidiol/.

45 Marissa Payne, "While Marijuana Remains Banned, WADA Reverses Course on Hemp-Derived Compound CBD," *Washington Post*, October 5, 2017, http://wapo.st/2geT4ho?tid=ss_tw&utm_term=.065a9fcc7dfa.

46 "Nate Diaz Vapes CBD Oil During His Post-UFC 202 Media Scrum," *Bleacher Report*, August 21, 2016, https://bleacherreport.com/articles/2658978-nate-diaz-vapes-cbd-oil-during-his-post-ufc-202-media-scrum.

47 Michelle Janikian, "CBD Is Allowed In The Olympics – How to Use CBD Like Olympians," Herb, Feb 19, 2018, https://herb.co/news/sports/olympians-allowed-use-cbd/.

48 Janet Burns, "WHO Report Finds No Public Health Risks Or Abuse Potential For CBD," *Forbes*, Mar 18, 2018, https://www.forbes.com/sites/janetwburns/2018/03/18/who-report-finds-no-public-health-risks-abuse-potential-for-cbd/.

49 World Health Organization, "Cannabidiol (CBD) Pre-Review Report Agenda Item 5.2," in *Expert Committee on Drug Dependence Thirty-Ninth Meeting*, Geneva, 2017.

50 Janet Burns, "Daily Dose Of Cannabis May Protect And Heal The Brain From Effects Of Aging," *Forbes*, May 8, 2017, https://www.forbes.com/sites/janetwburns/2017/05/08/daily-dose-of-cannabis-may-protect-and-heal-the-brain-from-effects-of-aging/#41dfc8652e44.

51 "For The Past 17 Years, Montel Williams Did What The FDA Won't: He Made Weed A Medicine," accessed February 13, 2019, https://www.forbes.com/sites/janetwburns/2017/04/20/for-17-years-montel-williams-has-been-perfecting-his-cannabis-line-now-its-ready/#263ff3cf792d.

Chapter Ten: Beyond CBD

52 Ethan B. Russo, "Beyond Cannabis: Plants and the Endocannabinoid System," *Trends in Pharmacological Sciences* 37, no. 7 (2016): 594–605, https://doi.org/10.1016/j.tips.2016.04.005.

53 "Boswellia: Uses, Dosage, Side Effects, and More," Healthline, October 23, 2013, https://www.healthline.com/health/boswellia.

54 "10 Health Benefits of Tart Cherry Juice," Healthline, June 10, 2017, https://www.healthline.com/nutrition/10-tart-cherry-juice-benefits.

55 "Bromelain: Dosage, Benefits, and Side Effects," Healthline, December 22, 2017, https://www.healthline.com/health/bromelain.

56 "Papain: Benefits, Side Effects, and More," Healthline, December 3, 2018, https://www.healthline.com/health/food-nutrition/papain.

57 "Serrapeptase: Uses, Side Effects, Interactions, Dosage, and Warning," WebMD, accessed February 13, 2019, https://www.webmd.com/vitamins/ai/ingredientmono-1115/serrapeptase.

58 "Cordyceps," *DrWeil.Com*, August 4, 2016, https://www.drweil.com/vitamins-supplements-herbs/herbs/cordyceps/.

59 "Jamaican Dogwood Herb Uses, Benefits, Cures, Side Effects, Nutrients," Herbpathy, accessed February 13, 2019, https://herbpathy.com/Uses-and-Benefits-of-Jamaican-Dogwood-Cid3264.

60 Adham M. Abdou et al., "Relaxation and Immunity Enhancement Effects of Gamma-Aminobutyric Acid (GABA) Administration in Humans," *BioFactors* (Oxford, England) 26, no. 3 (2006): 201–8.

61 "5-Htp: Uses, Side Effects, Interactions, Dosage, and Warning," WebMD, accessed February 13, 2019, https://www.webmd.com/vitamins/ai/ingredientmono-794/5-htp.

62 "California Poppy: Uses, Side Effects, Interactions, Dosage, and Warning," WebMD, accessed February 13, 2019, https://www.webmd.com/vitamins/ai/ingredientmono-104/california-poppy.

63 "Magnolia: Uses, Side Effects, Interactions, Dosage, and Warning," accessed February 13, 2019, https://www.webmd.com/vitamins/ai/ingredientmono-188/magnolia.

64 "Skullcap," Natural Medicines Professional Database, accessed February 13, 2019, https://naturalmedicines.therapeuticresearch.com/databases/food,-herbs-supplements/professional.aspx?productid=986.

65 National Center for Complementary and Integrative Health (NCCIH), Rhodiola factsheet (NCCIH Publication No. D492), https://nccih.nih.gov/health/rhodiola.

66 "Schisandra: Benefits, Side Effects, and Forms," Healthline, January 11, 2018, https://www.healthline.com/health/schisandra.

67 Jim English, "Beyond Ephedra: Bitter Orange (Citrus Aurantium)," *Nutrition Review*, April 19, 2013, https://nutritionreview.org/2013/04/beyond-ephedra-bitter-orange-citrus-aurantium/.

68 Arlene Semeco, "10 Benefits of Green Tea Extract," Healthline, July 22, 2017, https://www.healthline.com/nutrition/10-benefits-of-green-tea-extract.

69 Rena Goldman, "Ashwagandha: Benefits and Side Effects," Healthline, November 8, 2018, https://www.healthline.com/health/food-nutrition/ashwagandha-health-benefits.

70 Mayo Clinic Staff, "Milk Thistle," Mayo Clinic website, Oct. 14, 2017, https://www.mayoclinic.org/drugs-supplements-milk-thistle/art-20362885.

71 Elliott Almond, "Former NFL All-Pro Kyle Turley Now Fierce Advocate for Medical Marijuana," *The Cannabist*, September 8, 2017, https://www.thecannabist.co/2017/09/08/kyle-turley-marijuana-pharmaceuticals-painkillers-cte/87667/.

72 Gage Peak, "How Cannabis Helps UltraMarathoner Avery Collins Run 100 Miles," *Leafly*, August 4, 2016, https://www.leafly.com/news/lifestyle/how-cannabis-helps-ultramarathoner-avery-collins-run-100-miles.

73 Western States 100-Mile Endurance Run website, accessed February 13, 2019, https://www.wser.org/.

74 "Grindstone 100," Eco-Xsports website, accessed February 13, 2019, https://eco-xsports.com/events/grindstone-100/.

75 "The Indiana Trail 100," Ignite Trail Series website, accessed February 13, 2019, https://ignitetrailseries.com/indianatrail.html.

76 "Georgia Death Race," Run Bum Tours website, accessed February 13, 2019, https://www.runbumtours.com/georgia-death-race-1.

77 Frederick Dreier, "The Debate Over Running While High," *Wall Street Journal*, February 9, 2015, sec. Life, https://www.wsj.com/articles/the-debate-over-running-while-high-1423500590.